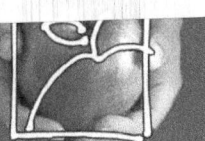

Food and Nutrition Information Center
National Agricultural Library USDA, 10301 Baltimore Ave., Room 105 Beltsville, MD 20705-2351

Food Allergies and Intolerances Resource List
for Consumers
December 2010

This publication is a collection of resources on the topic of Food Allergies and Intolerances for consumers. Resources include books, pamphlets, audiovisuals and Web sites. Many of the pamphlets are available in single copies and some may also be purchased in bulk from the organization listed (Web addresses are provided for materials available online). The books and audiovisuals can either be borrowed from your local library or purchased from your local book store.

Materials may also be borrowed from the National Agricultural Library (NAL) collection. Lending and copy service information is provided at the end of this document. If you are not eligible for direct borrowing privileges, check with your local library on how to borrow through interlibrary loan. Materials cannot be purchased from NAL. Contact information is provided for the producing organization if you wish to purchase or order any materials on this list. This contact information can be found in section C.

This Resource List is available from the Food and Nutrition Information Center's (FNIC) Web site at: http://www.nal.usda.gov/fnic/pubs/bibs/allergy.pdf. A complete list of FNIC publications can be found at http://fnic.nal.usda.gov/resourcelists.

Table of Contents

A. General Information on Food Allergies and Intolerances

1. Brochures and Fact Sheets

Do You Have a Food Allergy?
The Food Allergy & Anaphylaxis Network
Full text: http://www.foodallergy.org/files/DoYouHaveBrochure.pdf (PDF)
Description: Learn about the most common food allergens, symptoms of a food allergy and how food allergies are diagnosed.

Food Allergy: An Overview
National Institute of Allergy and Infectious Diseases, National Institutes of Health (NIH), U.S. Department of Health and Human Service (DHHS)
Full text: http://www.niaid.nih.gov/topics/foodAllergy/Documents/foodallergy.pdf (PDF)
Description: This pamphlet describes allergic reactions to foods and their possible causes and provides an overview of diagnosis and treatment methods for food allergies. It also describes other reactions to foods, known as food intolerances, which can be confused with food allergy, and discusses some unproven and controversial food allergy theories.
Ordering Information: NIH Publication No. 07-5518

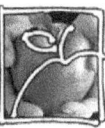

Tips to Remember - Food Allergies
American Academy of Allergy, Asthma and Immunology
Full text: http://www.aaaai.org/patients/publicedmat/tips/foodallergy.stm
http://www.aaaai.org/espanol/tips/alergias_a_los_alimentos.stm (Spanish)
Description: This brochure gives a basic overview of food allergies and intolerance, including the symptoms, diagnosis and treatment.
For a free single copy: http://www.aaaai.org/misc/inforequestform.stm
Online ordering: https://www.aaaai.org/patients/store/product.asp?productid=85

Understanding Food Allergy
International Food Information Council Foundation
Full text: http://www.foodinsight.org/Content/6/FINAL_Understanding-Food-Allergy_5-22-07.pdf (PDF)
Description: This brochure presents a summary of the key issues surrounding food allergies, including the definition, diagnosis and information for families of allergic individuals.
Online ordering: http://www.ificpubs.org/servlet/Detail?no=41

2. Books

Dealing with Food Allergies: A Practical Guide to Detecting Culprit Foods and Eating a Healthy, Enjoyable Diet
Janice Vickerstaff Joneja, PhD, RDN
Boulder, CO: Bull Publishing Company, 2003. 484 pp.
NAL Call Number: RC596.J665 2003
ISBN: 092352164X
Description: This book presents information on diagnostic methods and treatment options of food allergies and describes the effects of food allergies on the skin, mucous membranes and respiratory and digestive tracts. Content discusses treatment by allergists and other healthcare professionals and empowers readers to manage their food allergies.

Flourishing with Food Allergies: Social, Emotional and Practical Guidance for Families with Young Children
A. Anderson
Southbury, CT: Papoose Publishing, 2008. 360 pp.
ISBN: 0615187048
Description: This book includes stories from parents and guidance from medical professionals along with the latest research about food allergies. It includes discussions on shopping with food allergies in mind and advice on coping with food allergies at birthday parties, school and other venues. Suggestions are outlined for avoiding risky foods and re-thinking diet as well as creating a stress-free, safe-haven at home.

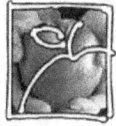

Food Allergies and Food Intolerance: A Complete Guide to Their Identification and Treatment
Johnathan Brostoff and Linda Gamlin
Rochester, VT: Healing Arts Press, 2000. 480 pp.
ISBN: 0892818751
Description: This book provides a comprehensive discussion on the difference between food allergies and food intolerance, including numerous case histories. Unique features include a detailed discussion of the controversy among the medical community concerning food intolerance and the effect it may contribute to conditions such as irritable bowl syndrome, rheumatoid arthritis, migraine headaches and others. The book provides a step-by-step process for diagnosing food intolerance using a 3-stage elimination diet and gradual food re-introduction. An appendix of foods with cross reactivity is also provided.

Food Allergy Survival Guide: Surviving and Thriving With Food Allergies and Sensitivities
Vesanto Melina, MS, RD, Jo Stepaniak, MSEd, and Dina Aronson, MS, RD
Summertown, TN: Healthy Living Publications, 2004. 383 pp.
NAL Call Number: RC596.M45 2004
ISBN: 157067163X
Description: This comprehensive resource offers a unique blend of scientific research, practical advice and culinary expertise. The book explains the differences between food allergy, food intolerance and food sensitivity; tests for allergies; how to avoid foods and ingredients that trigger reactions; how to maintain a healthy intestinal boundary; how to understand the latest food labeling regulations and how to create menus that meet special nutritional requirements.

How to Manage Your Child's Life-Threatening Food Allergies
Linda Marienhoff Coss
Lake Forest, CA: Plumtree Press, 2004. 208 pp.
NAL Call Number: RJ386.5 .C675 2004
ISBN: 0970278519
Description: This book provides step-by-step information to create a safe and enjoyable home, school and social environment for a child with food allergies. Topics covered include preparing for and treating allergic reactions, purchasing and cooking food, teaching others about food allergies, parenting issues, creating a safe school and day care environment, having a social life, dining in restaurants and traveling.

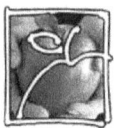

Let's Eat Out: Your Passport to Living Gluten and Allergy Free
Kim Koeller and Robert La France
R & R Publishing, 2005. 496 pp.
ISBN: 0976484501
Description: This full color book contains over 240 photos of delicious and savory foods. It explains options for eating out and includes 7 international cuisines outlining traditional ingredients, gluten awareness, allergy & dining considerations and sample menus. Also included are menu item descriptions and preparation requests, ingredient and preparation technique descriptions with sample questions to ask, snack and breakfast and beverage ideas and multi-lingual phrases.

Understanding and Managing Your Child's Food Allergies
Scott H. Sicherer
Baltimore, MD: The Johns Hopkins University Press, 2006. 336 pp.
ISBN: 0801884926
Description: This resource provides "emotional support and practical advice from a parent who's been there." The book describes why children develop food allergy, the symptoms of food allergy (affecting the skin, the gastrointestinal tract, and the respiratory system) and the role of food allergy in behavioral problems and developmental disabilities.

3. Cookbooks

Food Allergen-Free Baker's Handbook
Cybele Pascal
New York, NY: Celestial Arts. 2009. 200 pp.
ISBN: 1587613484
Description: This cookbook features recipes for baked goods, both sweet and savory, that omit the eight foods responsible for most allergies (milk, eggs, peanuts, tree nuts, fish, shellfish, soy and wheat). It requires stocking your pantry differently, but provides an extensive list of product resources.

Cooking Free: 200 Flavorful Recipes for People with Food Allergies and Multiple Food Sensitivities
Carol Fenster
New York, NY: Avery, 2005. 336 pp.
NAL Call Number: RC588.D53 F46 2005
ISBN: 1583332154
Description: This cookbook is comprised of recipes that remove four of the most common allergens--gluten, dairy, eggs and sugar--providing one book full of delicious recipes. The book includes recipes for breads, entrees, desserts and more, and is complete with food substitution and conversion tables.

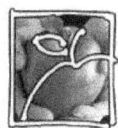

Flying Apron's Gluten-free & Vegan Baking Book
Jennifer Katzinger
Seattle, WA: Sasquatch Books, 2009. 192 pp.
ISBN: 1570616299
Description: Jennifer Katzinger, owner of the Flying Apron Bakery, shares her favorite sweet and savory, gluten-free, vegan recipes.

Great Foods without Worry
Cindy Mosely
Aventine Press, 2003. 164 pp.
ISBN: 1593301162
Description: "Great Foods Without Worry" offers a variety of recipes which omit wheat, eggs, dairy, soy, nuts and gluten. All recipes are suitable for vegetarian diets.

The Whole Foods Allergy Cookbook: Two Hundred Gourmet & Homestyle Recipes for the Food Allergic Family
Cybele Pascal
Ridgefield, CT: Vital Health Publishing, 2006. 213 pp.
NAL Call Number: RC588.D53 P368 2006
ISBN: 1890995223
Description: All recipes in this cookbook are free of the top eight allergens: dairy, eggs, wheat, soy, peanuts, tree nuts, fish or shellfish and also refined sugar. Baked goods are all vegan. Also included is a guide to gluten-free recipes, a shopping guide for hard-to-find items and a food allergy information resource guide.

4. Web Resources

Allergens
FoodSafety.gov, a cross-agency portal to food safety information from the U.S. Department of Agriculture and the U.S Department of Health and Human Service
Web site: http://www.foodsafety.gov/poisoning/causes/allergens/
Description: This cross-agency food safety site allows consumers to sign up for allergy alerts and has a link to a video on the differences between food allergies and intolerances.

Anaphylaxis
American Academy of Family Physicians
Web site: http://familydoctor.org/online/famdocen/home/common/allergies/basics/809.html
Description: This resource discusses anaphylaxis and what you need to know to prevent and treat it.

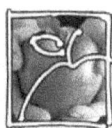

Breastfeeding & Allergies
La Leche League International
Web site: http://www.llli.org/NB/NBallergies.html
Description: This Web site provides multiple resources about allergies and the effect of breastfeeding on the development of food allergies.

Food Allergens
Food and Drug Administration (FDA), DHHS
Web site: http://www.fda.gov/Food/FoodSafety/FoodAllergens/default.htm
Description: This Web site provides information on food labeling and legislation related to food allergens.

Food Allergies
Asthma and Allergy Foundation of America
Web site: http://www.aafa.org/display.cfm?id=9&sub=20
Description: This Web site provides information on specific food allergies as well as a concise explanation of food allergies and related health issues.

Food Allergy
Mayo Foundation for Medical Education and Research
Web site: http://www.mayoclinic.com/health/food-allergy/DS00082
Description: This resource provides an overview of the signs and symptoms, causes and risk factors of food allergies. Information is also provided on when to seek medical advice, screening and diagnosis, treatment and prevention.

Food Allergy
National Institute of Allergy and Infectious Disease, NIH, DHHS
Web site: http://www.niaid.nih.gov/topics/foodallergy/pages/default.aspx
Description: This Web site includes quick facts, food allergy basics, news and events related to food allergies. Also included is a section on new research and a PDF report of the National Institute of Health Expert Panel on Food Allergy Research.

The Food Allergy and Anaphylaxis Network
The Food Allergy and Anaphylaxis Network
Web sites: http://www.foodallergy.org/
http://www.foodallergy.org/section/espanol (Spanish)
Description: FAAN offers many resources to parents and educators. This site offers management tips for the major food allergies as well as articles on other hot allergy issues. FAAN is the world's largest nonprofit organization providing patients information about food allergy and educational resources to schools, health professionals, restaurants, pharmaceutical companies and the food industry.

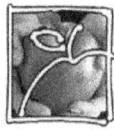

Food Allergy Initiative
Food Allergy Initiative
Web site: http://www.faiusa.org
Description: "The Food Allergy Initiative (FAI) is a 501 (c) (3) non-profit organization that raises funds toward the effective treatment and cure for food allergies." This organization's Web site includes information about food allergies and related issues, living with food allergies, information for food service providers, updates on research and public policy and facts sheets and press releases for media coverage.

Food Allergy Research and Resource Program
University of Nebraska-Lincoln
Web site: http://www.farrp.org
Description: This site contains allergen research, analysis, research, training opportunities and a workshop series. It also houses AllergenOnline, www.allergenonline.com, a peer reviewed allergen list and sequence searchable database intended for identifying proteins that may present a potential risk of allergenic cross-reactivity.

Physician Referral
American Academy of Allergy Asthma & Immunology
Web site: http://www.aaaai.org/physref/
Description: You enter a zip code or city and state and this Web site provides a list of asthma and allergy doctors in the area.

5. Resources for Children

Alexander Series
The Food Allergy and Anaphylaxis Network
Fairfax, VA: Food Allergy Network
Description: This children's series follows the daily life of Alexander, an elephant with a food allergy. The collection includes books, videos, DVDs, stuffed animals, stickers and more for elementary school-aged children. Books and resources include:
- A Special Day at School
- Alexander's First Babysitter
- Alexander's Special Holiday Treat
- Alexander Goes to a Birthday Party
- Alexander Goes Out to Eat
- Alexander's Fun & Games Activity Book
- Alexander Stuffed Animal
- Alexander, the Elephant Who Couldn't Eat Peanuts DVD **(NAL Call Number: Videocassette no. 2065)**

Online Ordering: https://www.foodallergy.org/members/msascart-ProductList?majorcat=featured&ONWEBFLG=Y&WHP=productHomeHeader.htm&WBP=productHomeList.htm

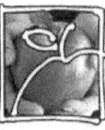

Allie the Allergic Elephant: A Children's Story of Peanut Allergies
Nicole Smith
Colorado Springs, CO: Allergic Child Publishing Group, 2006. 22 pp.
ISBN: 1586280538
Description: *Allie the Allergic Elephant* helps children learn about food allergies and how to be a good friend when you can't share snacks. Allie explains peanut allergies in a way that parents, teachers and children themselves can talk about allergies and understand them better.

Amy Goes Gluten Free: A Young Person's Guide to Celiac Disease
Children's Hospital Boston
Web site:
http://www.childrenshospital.org/clinicalservices/Site2166/mainpageS2166P0.html
Description: A fun comic book designed for children with activities and information to help learn about celiac disease.

Binky Goes Nuts: Understanding Peanut Allergies
PBS Kids
Web site: http://www.pbs.org/parents/arthur/lesson/health/#peanut
Description: The information and activities in this online activity unit help children learn how they can make their school a safe and healthy place for classmates who have peanut or other food allergies. This unit also includes a printable placemat with pictures and activities about peanut allergies.

The Bugabees: Friends with Food Allergies
Amy Recob
Minneapolis, MN: Beaver's Pond Press, 2009. 32 pp.
ISBN: 1592982794
Description: This book tells the story of eight friends with eight different food allergies: peanuts, tree nuts, fish, shellfish, milk, soy, eggs and wheat. Additional activities and talking points are included for parents and teachers.

Cody the Allergic Cow: A Children's Story of Milk Allergies
Nicole Smith
Jungle Communications, 2004. 26 pp.
ISBN: 1586280511
Description: This book teaches children and their friends, teachers and others to understand allergies to milk products.

A Day at the Playground with Food Allergies
Tracie Schrand
Llumina Kids, 2006. 26 pp.
ISBN: 1595266062
Description: This illustrated book offers young children some simple steps to avoid food allergens in a public place. Topics covered include sharing food, toys and hand washing.

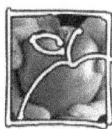

Food Allergies
Nemours Foundation
Web sites: http://www.kidshealth.org/kid/ill_injure/sick/food_allergies.html (kids)
http://www.kidshealth.org/teen/food_fitness/nutrition/food_allergies.html (teens)
Description: These two web resources provide informative articles about living with food allergies that are written for children and adolescents. The Web site also links to to more specific pages for children and teens about egg allergies, nut and peanut allergies, milk allergies and lactose intolerance. A printable diet card for each with a list of foods to avoid is included.

- Egg Allergies
  http://kidshealth.org/kid/nutrition/diets/egg_allergy.html (kids)
  http://kidshealth.org/teen/food_fitness/nutrition/egg_allergy.html (teens)
- Nut and Peanut Allergies
  http://kidshealth.org/kid/nutrition/diets/nut_allergy.html (kids)
  http://kidshealth.org/teen/food_fitness/nutrition/nut_allergy.html (teens)
- Lactose Intolerance:
  http://www.kidshealth.org/kid/health_problems/allergiesimmune/lactose.html (kids)
- Milk Allergy
  http://www.kidshealth.org/teen/nutrition/diets/milk_allergy.html (teens)

Food Allergies in the Real World
The Food Allergy & Anaphylaxis Network
Web site: http://www.faanteen.org/
Description: This Web site is designed for young adults who want to take a more active role in managing their food allergies.

Food Allergy News for Kids
The Food Allergy and Anaphylaxis Network
Web site: http://www.fankids.org/
Description: A Web site for kids to find out about food allergies, play games and activities, learn about different projects, ask questions and share stories about their food allergies.

Gluten-Free Friends: An Activity Book for Kids
Nancy Patin Falini
Centennial, CO: Savory Palate, Inc, 2003. 58 pp.
ISBN: 889374091
Description: This kids' coloring and activity book explains celiac disease and gluten intolerance. The book features Megan and Ben, two friendly kids who are following a gluten-free diet. Megan and Ben explain what gluten is in simple, non-technical words; describe how gluten makes kids with celiac disease get sick; decide which foods to avoid on a gluten-free diet and demonstrate how to make the right food choices to be healthy.

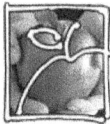

Lactose Intolerance
Office on Women's Health, DHHS
Web Site: http://www.girlshealth.gov/nutrition/lactose/index.cfm
Description: This Web site for teenage girls defines lactose intolerance and provides tips to help girls meet daily calcium requirements.

Mommy, Is this Safe to Eat? A Guide for Preschoolers Allergic to Peanuts and Tree Nuts
Christina Black
R3C Creations, LLC, 2006. 25pp.
ISBN: 1598723871
Description: This picture book teaches preschoolers with food allergies to always ask if a food is safe to eat.

No Lobster Please!
Robyn Rogers
Norfolk, MA: Heartsome Publishing, 2004. 30 pp.
ISBN: 0972640800
Description: This children's book tells a story about a boy with a severe and sensitive allergy to seafood.

Safe4Kids
Anaphylaxis Canada
Web site: www.safe4kids.ca
Description: A Web site for kids living with allergies and anaphylaxis. Resources include a gallery of artwork for children about food allergies, games and activities, recipes, stories, and a poster for schools.

Taking Food Allergies to School
Ellen Weiner
Valley Park, MO: JayJo Books, 1999. 32pp.
ISBN: 1891383051
Description: Written for children, this book includes topics such as sharing lunches, special parties and events and allergy-free snacks. A quiz for kids on food allergies and Ten Tips for Teachers (or parents) are provided.

You Must Be Nuts!
Kyle Dine
Web site: http://www.kyledine.com/
Description: This upbeat music CD delivers educational messages to children about food allergies. The CD contains 14 original tracks with names such as "Epi-Man," "Tingle on My Tongue," and "Gluten-Free Blues."
Online Ordering: http://www.kyledine.com/Purchase.htm

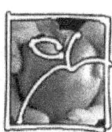

6. Other Resources

Food Allergy Among U.S. Children: Trends in Prevalence and Hospitalizations
National Center for Health Statistics, Centers for Disease Control and Prevention (CDC), DHHS
Full text: http://www.cdc.gov/nchs/data/databriefs/db10.pdf
Description: This data brief published in 2008 discusses the increase in prevalence of reported food allergy cases among children from 1997 to 2007.

Food Allergy Poster
International Food Information Council
Full text: http://internal.ific.org/publications/other/allergypos.cfm
http://internal.ific.org/publications/other/upload/FoodAllergyPoster.pdf (PDF)
Description: This poster was developed in cooperation with the American Academy of Allergy, Asthma and Immunology, the Food Allergy Network and the National Restaurant Association for food service workers. Available in both Spanish and English, the poster will help prepare food service workers to better identify and react to allergic reactions to food.

How to Read a Label Cards
The Food Allergy and Anaphylaxis Network
Description: These cards are designed to help families effectively read ingredient labels. Each wallet-sized, laminated card lists the various ways potential allergens can be listed on ingredient labels. Cards are available for milk, egg, peanut, wheat, tree nut, soy, and shellfish allergies.
Online Ordering: https://www.foodallergy.org/members/msascart-ProductList?majorcat=featured&ONWEBFLG=Y&WHP=productHomeHeader.htm&WBP=productHomeList.htm (select "Training Materials" and then scroll down to find the "How to Read a Label" card for the allergen you wish to avoid)

Kids with Food Allergies
Web site: www.kidswithfoodallergies.org
Description: "Kids with Food Allergies is a national nonprofit food allergy support group dedicated to fostering optimal health, nutrition, and well-being of children with food allergies…" This organization's Web site includes recipes, resources, and allergy alerts for kids with food allergies, their parents and other family members.

***Living Without* Magazine**
Web site: http://www.livingwithout.com
Description: *Living Without* is a quarterly magazine for people with allergies and food sensitivities. It discusses a variety of health-related issues, and provides support, encouragement, guidance and resources.
Online Ordering: http://www.livingwithout.com/subscribe.asp

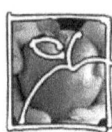

Support Forums
- AllergicChild.com: Food Allergy Support Group
  http://www.allergicchild.com/search_for_a_local_support_group.htm
- Kids With Food Allergies, Inc.: Parents of Food Allergic Kids Forum
  http://www.kidswithfoodallergies.org/community.html

Select Wisely
Web site: http://www.selectwisely.com/
Description: These wallet-sized cards contain food allergy messages and warnings in several foreign languages, which can be used when communicating with non-English speakers at home or abroad.

B.   Specific Allergies and Intolerances (in alphabetical order by allergen)

1. Egg

Egg Allergy
Cleveland Clinic Foundation
Web site:
http://my.clevelandclinic.org/childrens_hospital/pediatric_health_information/food_allergy_di
ets.aspx#2
Description: This fact sheet includes a chart that lists egg products, egg-containing ingredients and egg-containing foods. It also includes sample egg substitutions.

Egg Allergy Diet
Oregon Health and Science University
Web site: http://www.ohsu.edu/xd/health/health-information/topic-by-id.cfm?ContentTypeId=85&ContentId=P00015
Description: This Web article includes a comprehensive list of foods allowed and not allowed on an egg-free diet, categorized by food group. Also includes possible sources of eggs or egg products to look for on a food label and information for using egg substitutes.

Egg Allergy: The Facts
Allergy/Asthma Information Association of Canada
Full text: http://www.aaia.ca/en/egg_brochure_en.pdf (PDF 3KB)
http://www.aaia.ca/fr/egg_brochure_fr.pdf (French, PDF 5KB)
Description: This brochure explains what to look for on a food label, how to substitute for eggs in baking and reviews frequently asked questions.

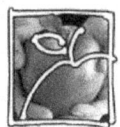

Nutrition and Fitness: Egg Allergy
Seattle Children's Hospital
Web site: http://www.seattlechildrens.org/kids-health/page.aspx?id=60795
Description: This Web site discusses how egg allergies are diagnosed and treated, and how an individual can live comfortably with an egg allergy.

Tips for Managing an Egg Allergy
The Food Allergy and Anaphylaxis Network
Web site: http://www.foodallergy.org/page/egg-allergy
Description: This online fact sheet provides substitutes for eggs when baking, identifies hidden sources of egg and answers common questions about egg allergies and influenza vaccines.

2. Fish and Shellfish

Fish Allergy
The Food Allergy & Anaphylaxis Network
Web site: http://www.foodallergy.org/page/fish-allergy
Description: This Web site lists unexpected sources of fish for allergic individuals to watch for, and answers frequently asked questions about food allergies.

Fish Allergy
Food Allergy Initiative
Web site: http://www.faiusa.org/?page=fish
Description: This web resource provides a simple description of fish allergies and lists foods that fish allergic individuals should avoid.

Seafood Allergy
Canadian Food Inspection Agency
ISBN: 978-1-100-14805-2
Full text: http://www.inspection.gc.ca/english/fssa/labeti/allerg/fispoie.shtml
http://www.inspection.gc.ca/english/fssa/labeti/allerg/fispoie.pdf (PDF 68KB)
Description: This brochure reviews the symptoms and treatment of seafood allergies, the difference between fish, crustacean and shellfish allergies, and histamine poisoning. It is also lists other names for fish, crustaceans and shellfish, possible food and nonfood sources.
Ordering Information: Cat. No. A104-84/2010E

Shellfish Allergy
Food Allergy Initiative
Web site: http://www.faiusa.org/?page=shellfish
Description: This web resource provides a simple description of fish allergies and lists foods that shellfish allergic individuals should avoid.

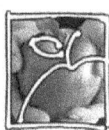

Shellfish Allergy
Mayo Foundation for Medical Education and Research
Web site: http://www.mayoclinic.com/health/shellfish-allergy/DS00987
Description: This web resource reviews signs and symptoms of a shellfish allergy, causes, screening and diagnosis, treatment and prevention.

3. Milk Allergies and Lactose Intolerance

Cow's Milk Allergy versus Lactose Intolerance
National Dairy Council
Full text:
http://www.nationaldairycouncil.org/Research/DairyCouncilDigestArchives/Pages/dcd77-3Page1.aspx
http://www.nationaldairycouncil.org/SiteCollectionDocuments/research/dairy_council_digests/2006/dcd773.pdf (PDF 322KB)
Description: This news article outlines the difference between milk protein allergy and lactose intolerance, including causes, prevalence, symptoms and management of each.

Milk Allergy
Food Allergy Initiative
Web site: http://www.faiusa.org/?page=milk
Description: This web article defines milk allergies and foods and ingredients to avoid. It also lists alternatives to milk and nondairy sources of calcium.

Milk Allergy
Mayo Foundation for Medical Education and Research
Web site: http://www.mayoclinic.com/health/milk-allergy/DS01008
Description: This substantial Web site includes information on milk allergy symptoms, causes, risk factors, complications, diagnosis, treatment, prevention and support.

Milk Allergy in Infants
Nemours Foundation
Web site: http://kidshealth.org/parent/medical/allergies/milk_allergy.html
Description: This comprehensive web article contains information specific to milk allergies in infants, including symptoms, diagnosis and treatment information, as well as unsafe formulas and advice for switching formulas.

Milk for Kids with Lactose Intolerance
Food and Nutrition Service, USDA
Web site: http://www.fns.usda.gov/tn/resources/nibbles/milk.pdf (PDF 10KB)
Description: This fact sheet for parents defines lactose intolerance, what to do if you suspect lactose intolerance in your child and how to incorporate milk products for a child who is lactose intolerant.

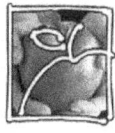

What I Need to Know About Lactose Intolerance
National Digestive Diseases Information Clearinghouse, National Institute of Diabetes and Digestive and Kidney Diseases (NIDDK), NIH, DHHS
Full text: http://digestive.niddk.nih.gov/ddiseases/pubs/lactoseintolerance_ez/
http://digestive.niddk.nih.gov/ddiseases/pubs/lactoseintolerance_ez/lactoseintolerance.pdf (PDF 30KB)
Description: An easy to read publication with colorful illustrations which outlines important points related to lactose intolerance, including symptoms of lactose intolerance, management of symptoms, identifying sources of lactose and getting enough calcium.
Ordering Information: NIH Publication No. 10-2751

What People with Lactose Intolerance Need to Know About Osteoporosis
National Institute of Arthritis and Musculoskeletal and Skin Diseases, National Institutes of Health (NIH) Osteoporosis and Related Bone Diseases ~ National Resource Center, NIH, DHHS
Full Text:
http://www.niams.nih.gov/health_info/bone/Osteoporosis/Conditions_Behaviors/lactose_intolerance.asp
http://www.niams.nih.gov/Health_Info/Bone/chinese/lactose_chinese.asp (Chinese)
Description: This web article defines the link between lactose intolerance and osteoporosis and provides bone health strategies to help strengthen bones when lactose intolerant.

4. Peanut / Tree Nut

Beyond a Peanut
Mind Flight LLC
Web site: http://www.beyondapeanut.com/
Description: These flashcards can be used to teach individuals about staying safe with a tree nut and peanut allergy.
Online Ordering: http://www.beyondapeanut.com/Beyond_A_Peanut_Products.html

The Complete Peanut Allergy Handbook
Scott H. Sicherer, MD and Terry Malloy
New York, NY: Berkeley Publishing Group, 2005. 304 pp.
ISBN: 0425204413
Description: This handbook is a guide to understanding and preventing peanut allergy attacks. Content includes information that parents need to know to protect themselves and their children from food allergies.

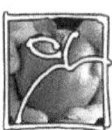

Flying with a Food Allergy
The Food Allergies and Anaphylaxis Network
Web site: http://www.foodallergy.org/page/7
Description: This online fact sheet provides guidelines for peanut-allergic airline passengers flying in the United States.

Peanut Allergy
Mayo Foundation for Medical Education and Research
Web site: http://www.mayoclinic.com/health/peanut-allergy/DS00710
Description: An article on peanut allergies that reviews the difference between peanut intolerances and peanut allergies, signs of an anaphylactic reaction, means of exposure and foods that can trigger symptoms. It also reviews risk factors, diagnosis and treatment options.

The Peanut Allergy Answer Book: 2nd Edition
Michael C. Young
New York, NY: Fair Winds Press, 2006. 168 pp.
ISBN: 1592332331
Description: Written by an allergist, this book provides the background medical information on peanut allergies, identifying peanut ingredients in foods, advice for dealing with schools, daycare centers and airlines.

Tree Nuts - One of the Nine Most Common Food Allergens
Canadian Food Inspection Agency
Catalogue No.: A104-84/2010E
ISBN: 978-1-100-14805-2
Full text: http://www.inspection.gc.ca/english/fssa/labeti/allerg/nutnoie.shtml
http://www.inspection.gc.ca/english/fssa/labeti/allerg/nutnoie.pdf (PDF 10KB)
Description: This brochure reviews symptoms and treatment options for tree nut allergies, as well as frequently asked questions about tree nut allergies.

5. Sesame Seeds

Seed Allergy
Food Allergy Initiative
Web site: http://www.faiusa.org/?page=seeds
Description: This Web site contains information about how to avoid eating sesame seeds, and includes a list of ingredients and foods that indicate the presence of sesame seed protein.

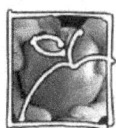

Sesame Allergy Facts
Kids with Food Allergies
Web site:
http://www.kidswithfoodallergies.org/resourcespre.php?id=107&title=sesame_allergy
Description: Web article on the growth of sesame seed allergies in children.

Sesame seeds - One of the nine most common food allergens
Canadian Food Inspection Agency
Full text: http://www.inspection.gc.ca/english/fssa/labeti/allerg/sese.shtml
http://www.inspection.gc.ca/english/fssa/labeti/allerg/sese.pdf (PDF 4KB)
Description: This brochure reviews symptoms and treatment of an allergic reaction and
frequently asked questions about sesame seed allergies.

6. Soy

Soy Allergy
Cleveland Clinic Foundation
Web site: http://www.clevelandclinic.org/health/health-info/docs/3300/3322.asp?index=11320
Description: This article provides information on who gets soy allergies, what are the
symptoms, how to avoid exposure and how to be prepared for a reaction.

Soy Allergy
Mayo Foundation for Medical Education and Research
Web site: http://www.mayoclinic.com/health/soy-allergy/DS00970
Description: A Web article that reviews the signs of a soy allergy, causes, risk factors and
products to avoid, including hidden sources of soy.

Tips for Managing a Soy Allergy
The Food Allergy and Anaphylaxis Network
Web site: http://www.foodallergy.org/allergens/soy.html
Description: This Web site includes three quick tips for people with soy allergies, a soy-
free recipe and links to an article about the relationship between peanut and soy allergies.

7. Sulfite Sensitivity

Sulfite Sensitivity
Canadian Food Inspection Agency
Full text: http://www.inspection.gc.ca/english/fssa/labeti/allerg/sulphe.shtml
http://www.inspection.gc.ca/english/fssa/labeti/allerg/sulphe.pdf (PDF 1KB)
Description: This brochure answers frequently asked questions about sulphite sensitivity.
It also includes lists of alternate names for sulphite, food and nonfood sources and tips to
prevent cross-contamination.

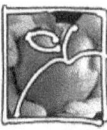

Sulfite Sensitivity
Cleveland Clinic Foundation
Web site:
http://my.clevelandclinic.org/disorders/sulfite_sensitivity/hic_sulfite_sensitivity.aspx
Description: This article gives an overview of where sulfites are found, symptoms of a sulfite allergy, and how it is diagnosed.

Sulfites
Food Marketing Institute
Web site: http://www.fmi.org/media/bg/?fuseaction=sulfites
Description: This web article defines what sulfites are and how they are used in food. It describes how to detect sulfites on food labels and lists food sources of sulfites.

8. Wheat/Gluten Allergy and Sensitivity

Celiac Disease
American Celiac Disease Alliance
Web site: http://americanceliac.org/celiac-disease/
http://americanceliac.org/celiac-disease/cd-spanish/ (Spanish)
Description: This web article discusses the difference between wheat allergy, gluten intolerance and celiac disease.

Celiac Disease News
Celiac Disease Awareness Campaign
Full Text: http://www.celiac.nih.gov/Newsletter.aspx
Description: This email newsletter features news about celiac disease, special events, patient and professional meetings and new publications. Available in html and PDF format.
Online Ordering: http://www.celiac.nih.gov/NewsletterSubscription.aspx

Celiac Disease Nutrition Guide, 2nd Edition
Tricia Thompson, MS, RD
Chicago, IL: American Dietetic Association, 2006. 48 pp.
ISBN: 0880913061
Web site: http://www.eatright.org/Shop/Product.aspx?id=5052
Description: This edition "survival guide" provides essential information for people diagnosed with Celiac disease.
Ordering Information: Order online from the American Dietetic Association call 1-800-877-1600 ext. 5000.

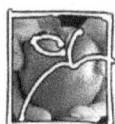

Gluten Free Diet Guide for Families
Children's Digestive Health and Nutrition Foundation
Full text: http://www.cdhnf.org/user-assets/documents/pdf/GlutenFreeDietGuideWeb.pdf
(PDF 6 KB)
http://www.cdhnf.org/user-assets/documents/pdf/GlutenFreeDietGuideWebSpanish.pdf
(Spanish, PDF 196KB)
Description: This booklet is a starter guide for newly diagnosed celiac patients and their families. The topics cover where gluten is found, what patients can eat, a shopping guide and more.

Gluten Intolerance Group Publications
Gluten Intolerance Group of North America
Full text: http://www.gluten.net/publications.php
Description: A variety of consumer-friendly articles, brochures, recipes and other resources on topics related to celiac disease. All publications may be downloaded free of charge in PDF file format. Some resources are available in Spanish.

Quick Start Diet Guide for Celiac Disease
Celiac Disease Foundation, Gluten Intolerance Group
Full text: http://www.gluten.net/downloads/print/QuickStartDiet.pdf (PDF 385 KB)
Description: This educational bulletin explains what is allowed and not allowed on a gluten free diet, what to look for on food labels and how to adjust to a new diet.

Raising Your Celiac Child
Children's Hospital Boston
Web site:
http://www.childrenshospital.org/clinicalservices/Site2166/mainpageS2166P12.html
Description: This 12-segment video resource was developed to help families learn more about managing celiac disease. The video topics are varied and include how to start and maintain a gluten free diet, how to eat out at school and restaurants, how to adjust & cope emotionally and more. Individual segments of the DVD can be viewed online or the entire DVD can be ordered.

What I Need to Know About Celiac Disease
National Digestive Diseases Information Clearinghouse, National Institute of Diabetes, Digestive and Kidney Diseases (NIDDK), NIDDK, NIH, DHHS
Full text: http://digestive.niddk.nih.gov/ddiseases/pubs/celiac_ez/index.htm
http://digestive.niddk.nih.gov/ddiseases/pubs/celiac_ez/WINTKACeliacDisease.pdf (PDF)
http://digestive.niddk.nih.gov/spanish/pubs/celiac_ez/index.htm (Spanish)
Description: An easy-to-read booklet defining celiac disease and outlining its symptoms, diagnosis and treatment. The booklet includes some examples of a gluten-free diet.
Ordering Information: NIH Publication No. 07-5755
Online Ordering: http://catalog.niddk.nih.gov/detail.cfm?ID=899

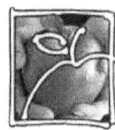

Wheat Allergy
The Food Allergy and Anaphylaxis Network
Web site: http://www.foodallergy.org/page/wheat-allergy
Description: This Web site answers frequently asked questions about wheat allergies, including the difference between celiac disease and wheat allergy, and how to substitute for wheat flour when baking.

Wheat Allergy
Mayo Foundation for Medical Education and Research
Web site: http://www.mayoclinic.com/health/wheat-allergy/DS01002
Description: This article reviews most aspects of a wheat allergy, including symptoms, causes, risk factors, diagnosis, treatment and prevention. The article includes a list of hidden sources of wheat products and tips for eating out.

Wheat Allergy Information
Food Allergy Initiative
Web site: http://www.faiusa.org/?page=wheat
Description: This Web site defines wheat allergy, and provides a list of common names of wheat and foods containing wheat to avoid. It also lists wheat-free alternatives to explore.

9. Other Allergies and Sensitivities

Corn Allergies
Children's Hospital for the King's Daughters
Web site: http://www.chkd.org/HealthLibrary/Facts/Content.aspx?pageid=0458
Description: This Web site lists foods that are likely to have corn products, ingredients that may indicate a presence of corn and foods to use vs. foods to avoid.

Food Additives
Asthma and Allergy Foundation of America
Web site: http://www.aafa.org/display.cfm?id=9&sub=20&cont=285
Description: This Web site explains adverse reactions to food additives, possible symptoms, diagnosis and prevention. It also lists and defines the eight most common food additives that may cause reactions.

Oral Allergy Syndrome
Allergy UK, British Allergy Foundation
Web site: http://www.allergyuk.org/fs_oralallergy.aspx
Description: This Web site includes symptoms, causes and management of oral allergy syndrome. Also includes a chart comparing recognized associations between pollen and food allergies

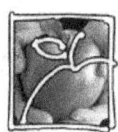

C. Contact Information for Organizations Cited (in alphabetical order)

Allergy/Asthma Information Association of Canada
295 The West Mall, Suite 118
Toronto, ON M9C 4Z4
Phone: 1-800-611-7011 or 416-621-4571   Fax: 416-621-5034
E mail: admin@aaia.ca
Web site: http://aaia.ca/en/index.htm

Allergy UK, British Allergy Foundation
Planwell House
LEFA Business Park
Edgington Way
Sidcup, Kent
DA14 5BH
Phone: 01322 619898
Email: info@allergyuk.org
Web site: http://www.allergyuk.org

American Academy of Allergy, Asthma & Immunology
555 East Wells Street, Suite 1100
Milwaukee, WI 53202-3823
Phone: 800-822-2762 or 414-272-6071
Email: info@aaaai.org
Web site: http://www.aaaai.org/

American Academy of Family Physicians
P.O. Box 11210
Shawnee Mission, KS 66207-1210
Phone: 800-274-2237
Email: contactcenter@aafp.org
Web site: http://www.aafp.org/

American Celiac Disease Alliance
2504 Duxbury Place
Alexandria, VA 22308
Phone: (703) 622-3331
Email: info@americanceliac.org
Web site: http://americanceliac.org/

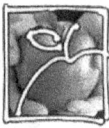

Anaphylaxis Canada
2005 Sheppard Avenue East, Suite 800
Toronto, Ontario M2J 5B4
Canada
Phone: 416-785-5666   Fax: 416-785-0458
Email: info@anaphylaxis.ca
Web site: http://www.anaphylaxis.org/

Asthma and Allergy Foundation of America
1233 20th Street, NW, Suite 402
Washington, DC 20036
Phone: 800-7-ASTHMA (800-727-8462)
Email: Info@aafa.org
Web site: http://www.aafa.org/

Beyond A Peanut
Phone: 720-482-0384
Email: info@beyondapeanut.com
Web site: http://beyondapeanut.com

Canadian Food Inspection Agency
Phone: 1-800-442-2342
Email: http://www.inspection.gc.ca/english/tools/feedback/commene.shtml
Web site: http://www.inspection.gc.ca/

Celiac Disease Awareness Campaign
c/o National Digestive Diseases Information Clearinghouse
2 Information Way
Bethesda, MD 20892–3570
Phone: 800–891–5389   Fax: 703–738–4929
Email: celiac@info.niddk.nih.gov
Web site: www.celiac.nih.gov

Celiac Disease Foundation
13251 Ventura Blvd. #1
Studio City, Ca. 91604
Phone: 818-990-2354   Fax: 818-990-2379
Email: cdf@celiac.org
Web site: http://www.celiac.org/

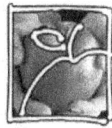

Celiac Sprue Association/United States of America, Inc.
P.O. Box 31700
Omaha, NE 68131-0700
Phone: 877-CSA-4-CSA (877-272-4272) or 402-558-0600
Email: celiacs@csaceliacs.org
Web site: www.csaceliacs.org

Center for Disease Control and Prevention (CDC)
1600 Clifton Rd.
Atlanta, GA 30333
Phone: 800-232-4636
Email: cdcinfo@cdc.gov
Web site: http://www.cdc.gov/

Center for Food Safety and Applied Nutrition
Food and Drug Administration
CFSAN Outreach and Information Center
5100 Paint Branch Parkway HFS-009
College Park, MD 20740-3835
Phone: 800-SAFEFOOD (800-723-3366)
Web site: http://www.fda.gov/Food/default.htm

Children's Digestive Health and Nutrition Foundation
1501 Bethlehem Pike
P. O. Box 6
Flourtown, PA 19031
Phone: 215-233-0808
Email: cdhnf@cdhnf.org
Web site: http://www.cdhnf.org/

Children's Hospital Boston
Children's Hospital Celiac Support Group c/o
Division of Gastroenterology and Nutrition
300 Longwood Avenue
Boston, MA 02115
Phone: 617-355-6000
Web site: http://www.childrenshospital.org/

Children's Hospital of the King's Daughters
601 Children's Lane
Norfolk, VA 23507
Phone: 757-668-7000
Email: http://chkd.org/Contact.aspx
Web site: http://chkd.org/

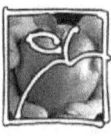

Cleveland Clinic Foundation
Cleveland Clinic
9500 Euclid Avenue
Cleveland, OH 44195
Phone: 800.223.2273 ext. 55580
Web site: http://www.clevelandclinic.org/

***FDA Consumer* Magazine**
Food and Drug Administration
5600 Fishers Lane, Room 15A-29
Rockville, MD 20857
Phone: 1-888-INFO-FDA (1-888-463-6332)
Web site: http://www.fda.gov/FDAC/
For more information on print orders, please see:
http://www.fda.gov/opacom/catalog/order.html

The Food Allergy and Anaphylaxis Network
11781 Lee Jackson Hwy., Suite 160
Fairfax, VA 22033-3309
Phone: 800-929-4040   Fax: 703-691-2713
Email: http://www.foodallergy.org/page/contact
Web site: http://foodallergy.org/

Food Allergy Initiative
1414 Avenue of the Americas, Suite 1804
New York, NY 10019
Phone: 212-207-1974   Fax: 917-338-5130
Email: info@faiusa.org
Web site: http://www.faiusa.org/

Food Allergy Research and Resource Program
143 Food Industry Complex
University of Nebraska
Lincoln, NE 68583-0919
Phone: 402-472-2833 (Steve Taylor, Ph.D.)   Fax: 402-472-5307
Email: farrp@unl.edu
Web site: http://farrp.org/

Food and Drug Administration
10903 New Hampshire Ave.
Silver Spring, MD 20993
Phone: 888-463-6332
Email: webmail@oc.fda.gov
Web site: http://www.fda.gov/

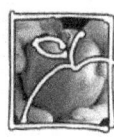

Food and Nutrition Service
U.S. Department of Agriculture
3101 Park Center Drive
Alexandria, VA 22302
Phone: 703-305-2062
Web site: http://www.fns.usda.gov/fns/

Food Marketing Institute
2345 Crystal Drive, Suite 800
Arlington, VA 22202
Phone: 202-452-8444
Email: http://www.fmi.org/?fuseaction=contact
Website: http://www.fmi.org/

Food Safety and Inspection Service
U.S. Department of Agriculture
1400 Independence Ave., S.W.
Washington, DC 20250-3700
Phone: 800-233-3935
Email: http://www.fsis.usda.gov/contact_us/Electronic_Mailboxes_Available/index.asp
Website: http://www.fsis.usda.gov/

Gluten Intolerance Group of North America
31214 124th Ave SE
Auburn,WA 98092-3667
Phone: 253-833-6655   Fax: 253-833-6675
Email: info@gluten.net
Web site: www.gluten.net

International Food Information Council Foundation
1100 Connecticut Avenue, N.W., Suite 430
Washington, DC 20036
Phone: 202-269-6540   Fax: 202-269-6547
Email: info@foodinsight.org
Web site: http://www.foodinsight.org/

Kids with Food Allergies
73 Old Dublin Pike, Ste 10, #163
Doylestown, PA 18901
Phone: 215-230-5394   Fax: 215-340-7674
Email: http://www.kidswithfoodallergies.org/email.php?to=info
Web site: http://www.kidswithfoodallergies.org/

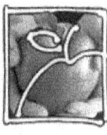

La Leche League International
PO Box 4079
Schaumburg, IL 60168-4079
Phone: 1-800-LaLeche (800-525-3243)   Fax: 847-969-0460
Email: http://www.llli.org/contact/contact_us
Web site: http://www.llli.org/

Living Without **Magazine**
PO Box 1998
Sun Valley, Idaho 83353
Web site: http://www.livingwithout.com

Mayo Foundation for Medical Education and Research
Email: http://www.mayoclinic.com/health/contact-us/contactus
Web site: http://www.mayoclinic.com/

National Dairy Council
10255 W. Higgins Rd., Suite 900
Rosemont, IL 60018
Email: http://www.nationaldairycouncil.org/AboutNDC/Pages/ContactUs.aspx
Web site: http://www.nationaldairycouncil.org/

National Digestive Diseases Information Clearinghouse
National Institute of Diabetes, Digestive and Kidney Diseases (NIDDK), National Institutes of Health
NIDDK Clearinghouses Publications Catalog
5 Information Way
Bethesda, MD 20892–3568
Phone: 800–860–8747   Fax: 703–738–4929
Email: catalog@niddk.nih.gov
Web site: http://catalog.niddk.nih.gov/

National Institute of Allergy and Infectious Disease
National Institutes of Health
NIAID News and Public Information Branch
6610 Rockledge Drive, MSC 6612
Bethesda, MD 20892-6612
Phone: 866-284-4107   Fax: 301-402-3573
E-mail: http://www3.niaid.nih.gov/links_policies/contact_us.htm
Web site: http://www.niaid.nih.gov/

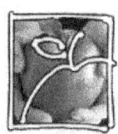

National Institute of Arthritis and Musculoskeletal and Skin Diseases
National Institutes of Health
1 AMS Circle
Bethesda, MD 20892-3675
Phone: 301-495-4484; 877-226-4267
Email: NIAMSinfo@mail.nih.gov
Website: http://www.niams.nih.gov

Nemours Foundation
Email (Kid's Health): comments@KidsHealth.org
Web site: http://www.nemours.org/
Web Site (Kid's Health): http://www.kidshealth.org/index.html

Office on Women's Health
U. S. Department of Health and Human Services
Phone: 800-994-9662
Email: http://www.womenshealth.gov/contact/index.cfm?sawquestions=yes
Websites: http://www.womenshealth.gov/ ; http://www.girlshealth.gov/

Oregon Health and Sciences University
3181 S.W. Sam Jackson Park Rd.
Portland, Oregon 97239-3098
Phone: 503-494-5274
Email: http://www.ohsu.edu/xd/about/contact.cfm
Website: http://www.ohsu.edu/xd/

PBS Kids
Email: http://www.pbs.org/parents/feedback.html
Web site: http://pbskids.org/

Seattle Children's Hospital
4800 Sand Point Way NE
Seattle, WA 98105
Phone: 206-987-2000
Email: http://www.seattlechildrens.org/about/contact-form/
Web site: http://www.seattlechildrens.org/

Select Wisely
PO Box 289
2 Main Street
Sparta, New Jersey 07871 USA
Phone: 888-396-9260
Email: orders@selectwisely.com
Web site: http://www.selectwisely.com/

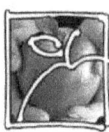

This resource list was compiled by:
Lorraine Butler, RD, Nutrition Information Specialist
Rachel Tobin, MS, RD, Nutrition Information Specialist

Acknowledgment is given to the following FNIC reviewer:
Gina Hundley Gomez, RD, Nutrition Information Specialist

This publication was developed in part through a Cooperative Agreement with the Department of Nutrition and Food Science in the College of Agriculture and Natural Resources at the University of Maryland.

Locate additional FNIC publications at http://fnic.nal.usda.gov/resourcelists.

Food and Nutrition Information Center
Agricultural Research Service, USDA
National Agricultural Library, Room 105
10301 Baltimore Avenue
Beltsville, MD 20705-2351
Phone: 301-504-5414
Fax: 301-504-6409
TTY: 301-504-6856
Contact: http://fnic.nal.usda.gov/contact
Web site: http://fnic.nal.usda.gov

The National Agricultural Library (NAL) provides lending and photocopying services to U.S. Department of Agriculture (USDA) employees. Non-USDA users can obtain materials from NAL through the interlibrary lending services of their local, corporate, or university library. For further information on NAL's document delivery services visit their Web site at http://www.nal.usda.gov/services/request.shtml.

For questions on document delivery services please call 301-504-5717 or submit a question at http://www.nal.usda.gov/services/ask.php.

The use of trade, firm, or corporation names in this publication (or page) is for the information and convenience of the reader. Such use does not constitute an official endorsement or approval by the USDA or the Agricultural Research Service (ARS) of any product or service to the exclusion of others that may be suitable.

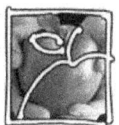

USDA prohibits discrimination in all its programs and activities on the basis of race, color, national origin, age, disability, and where applicable, sex, marital status, familial status, parental status, religion, sexual orientation, genetic information, political beliefs, reprisal, or because all or a part of an individual's income is derived from any public assistance program. (Not all prohibited bases apply to all programs.)

Persons with disabilities who require alternative means for communication of program information (Braille, large print, audiotape, etc.) should contact USDA's TARGET Center at 202-720-2600 (voice and TDD).

To file a complaint of discrimination write to USDA, Director, Office of Civil Rights, 1400 Independence Avenue, S.W., Washington, D.C. 20250-9410 or call 800-795-3272 (voice) or 202-401-0216 (TDD). USDA is an equal opportunity provider and employer.

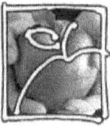